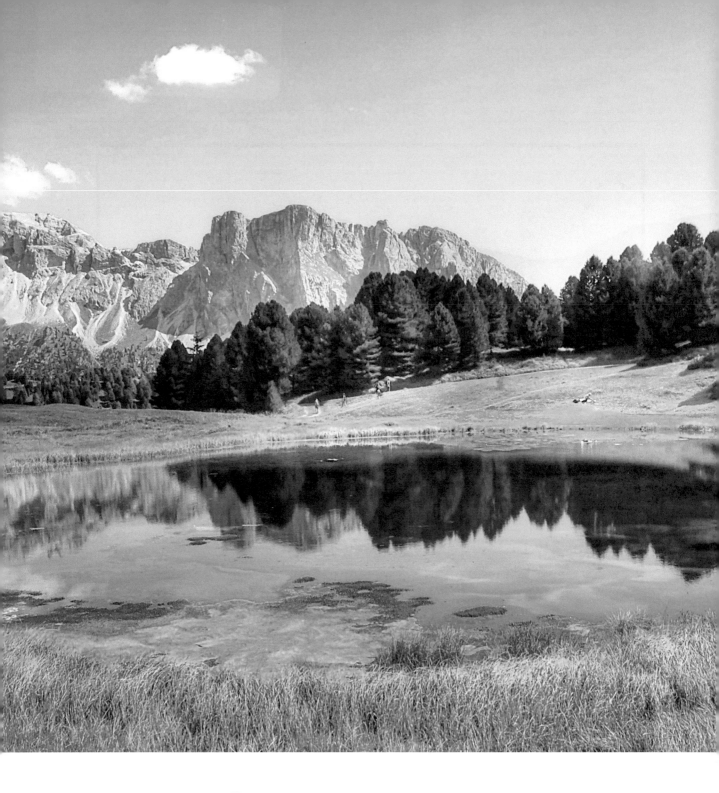

Serene

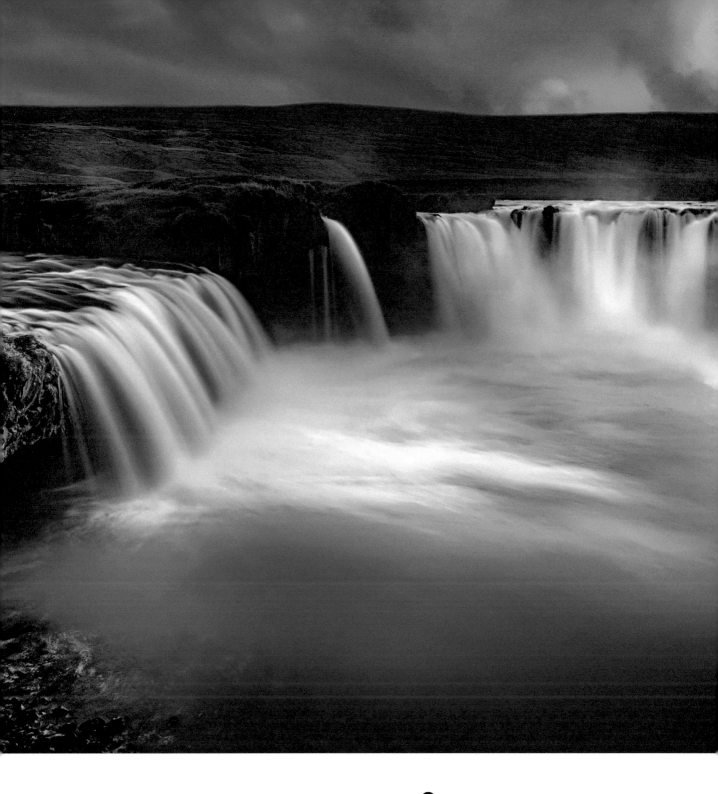

Stunning

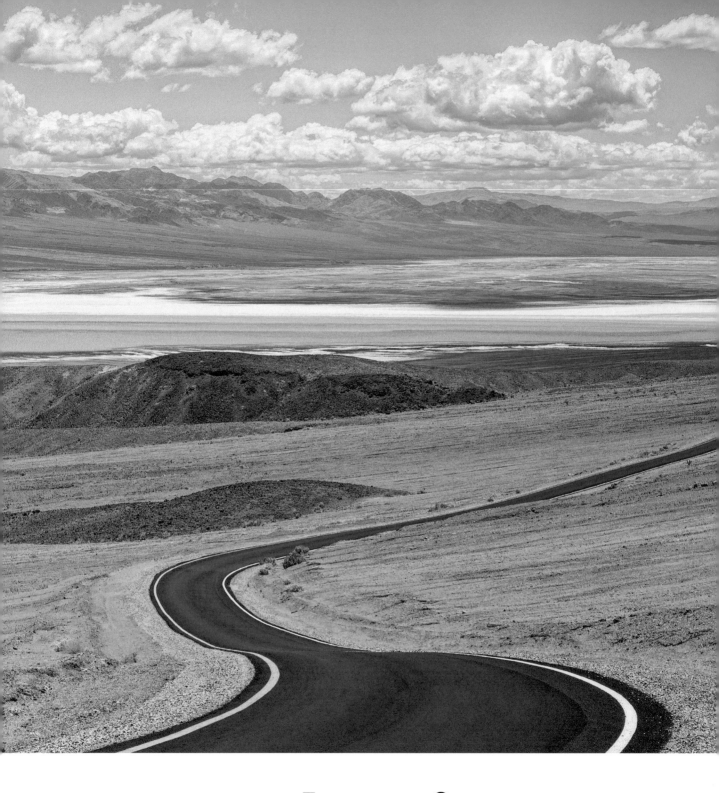

Relaxing

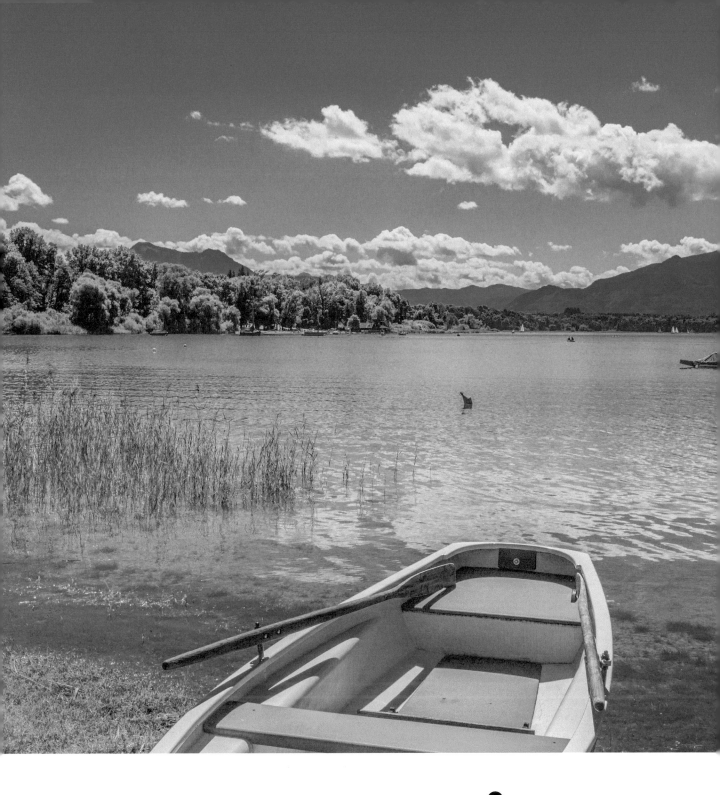

Fantastic

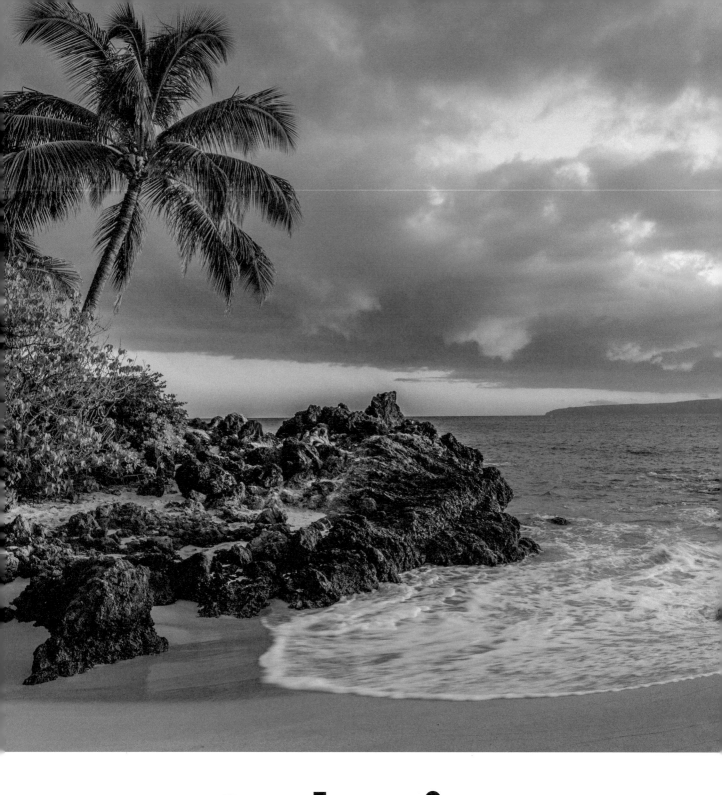

Calming

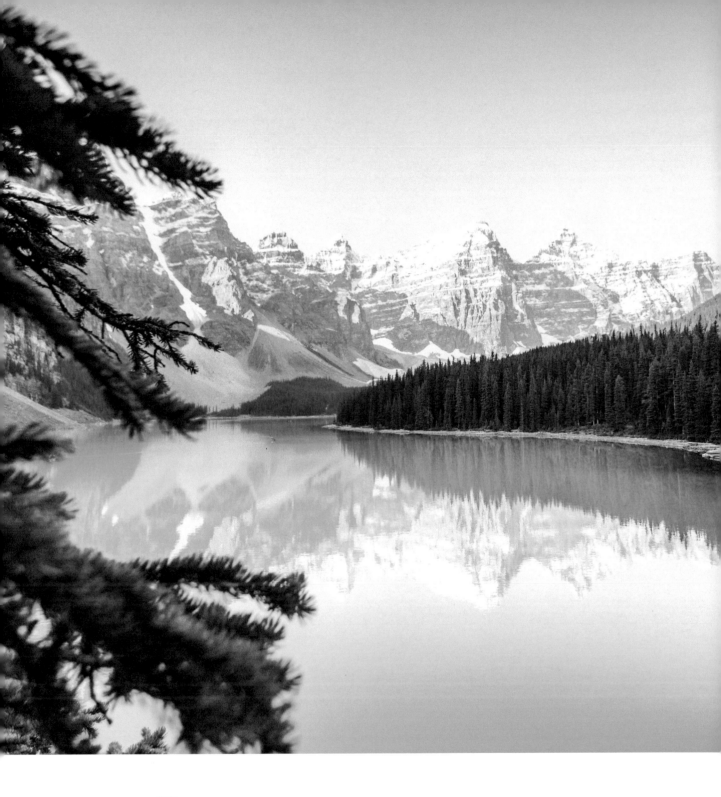

Gorgeous

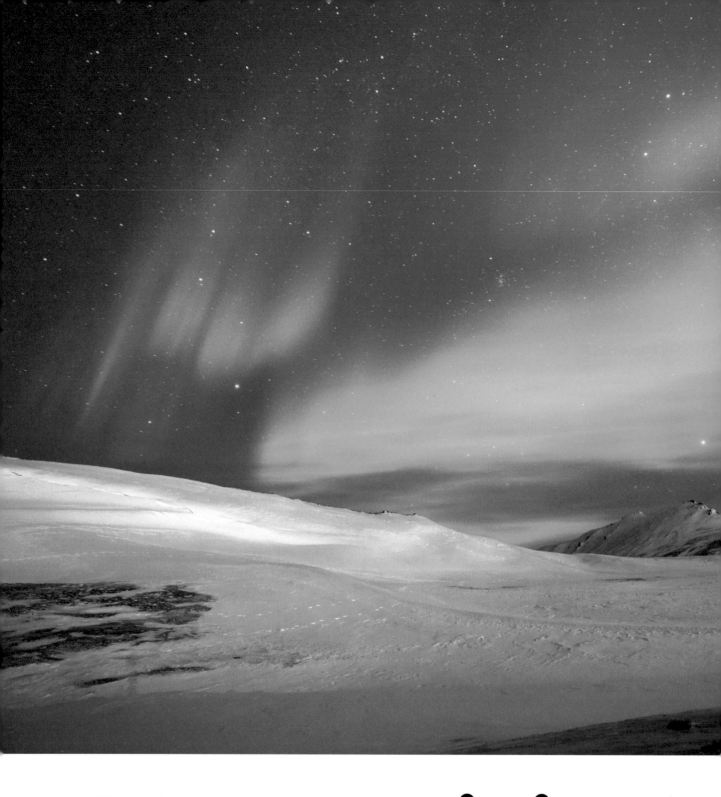

Mesmerizing

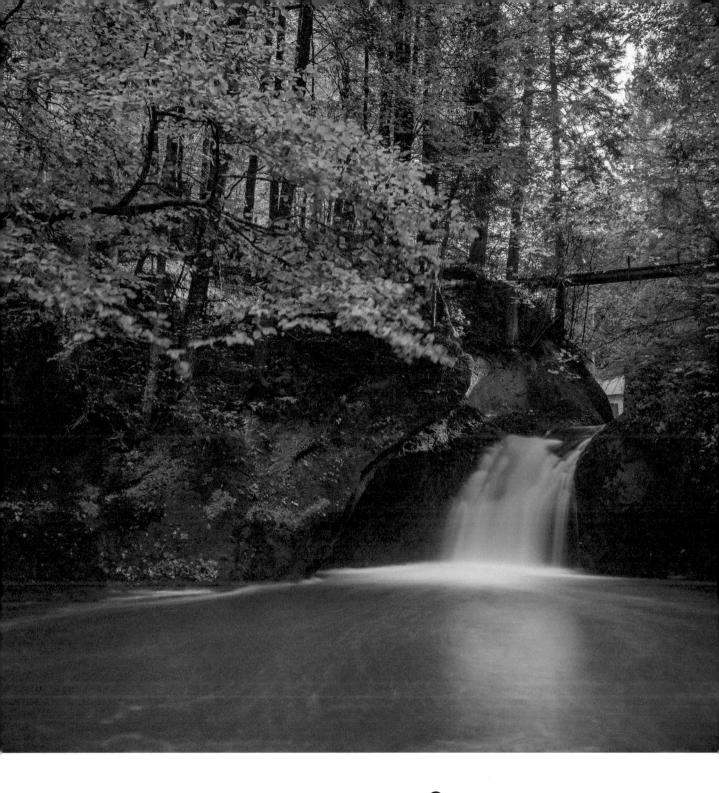

Scenic

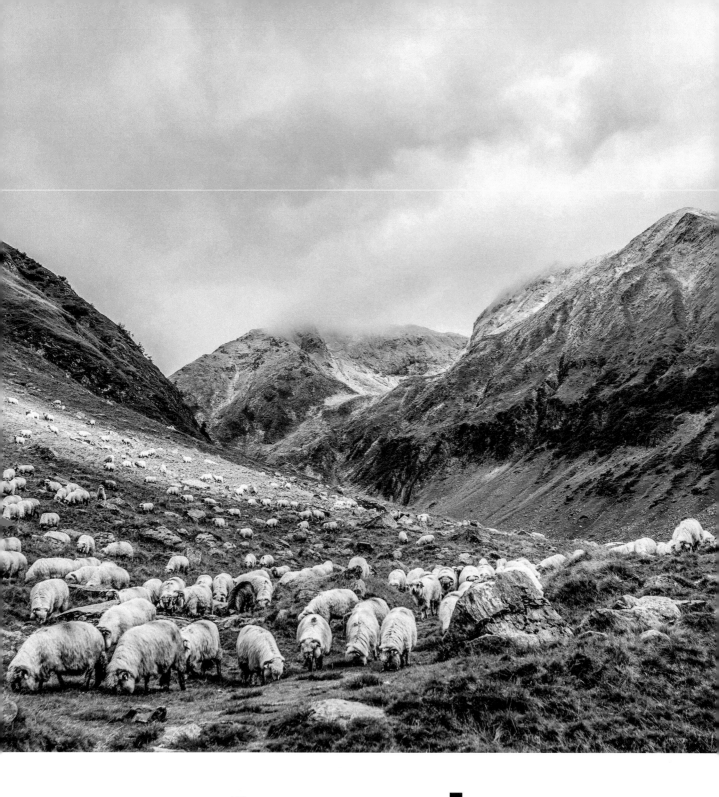

Lovely

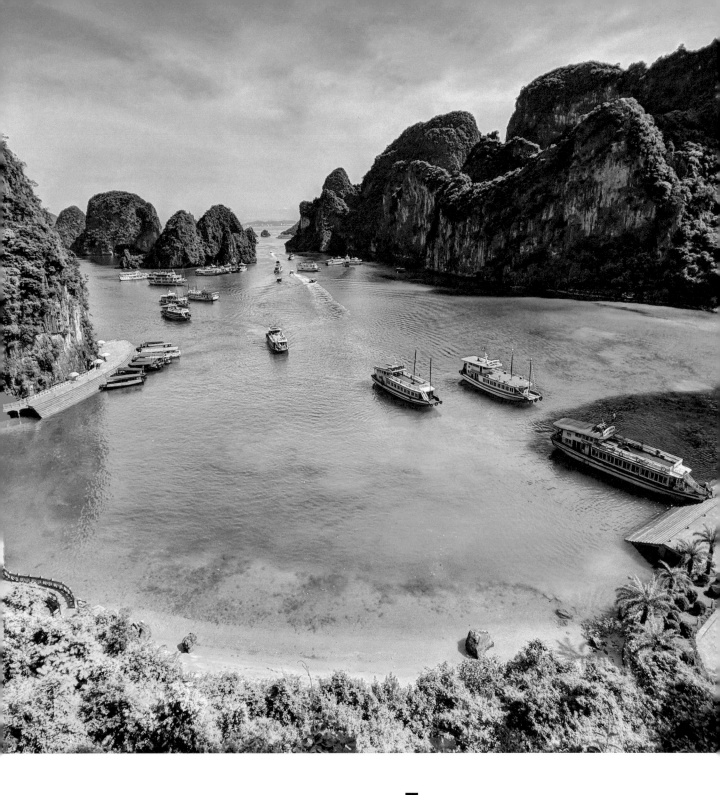

Marvelous

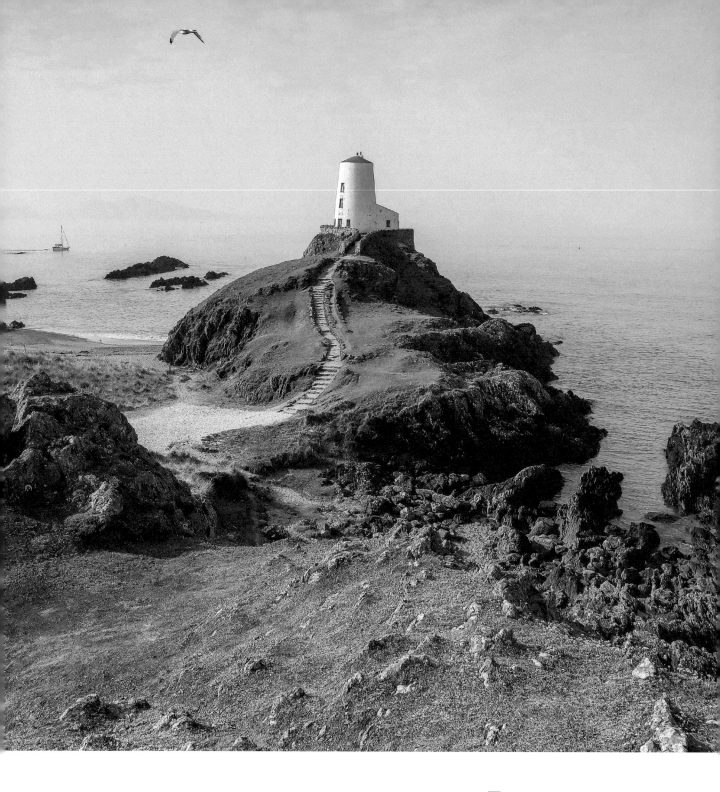

Superb

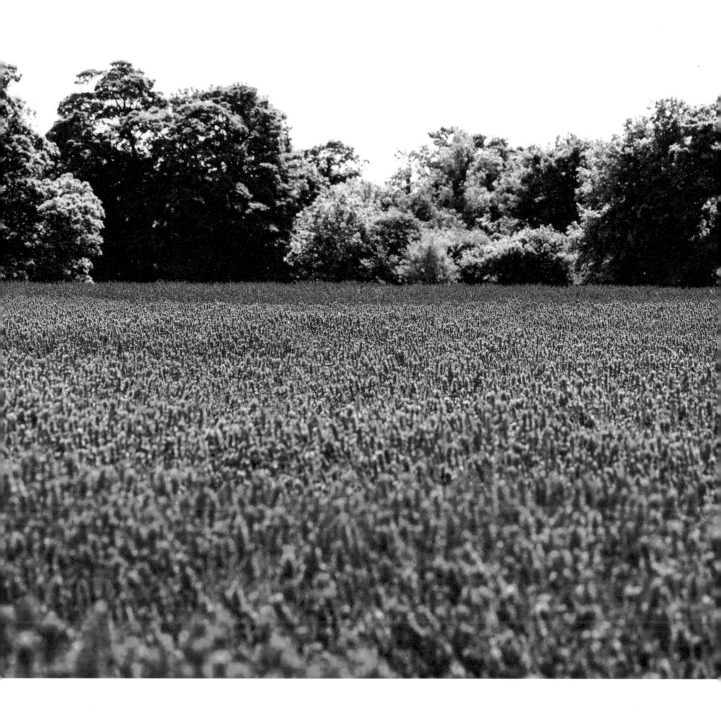

Tranquil

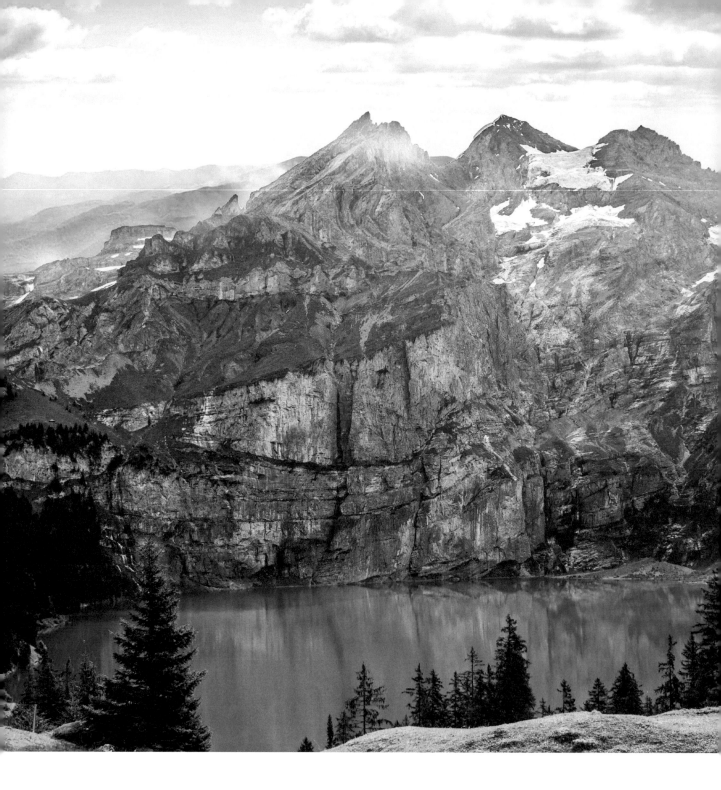

Peaceful

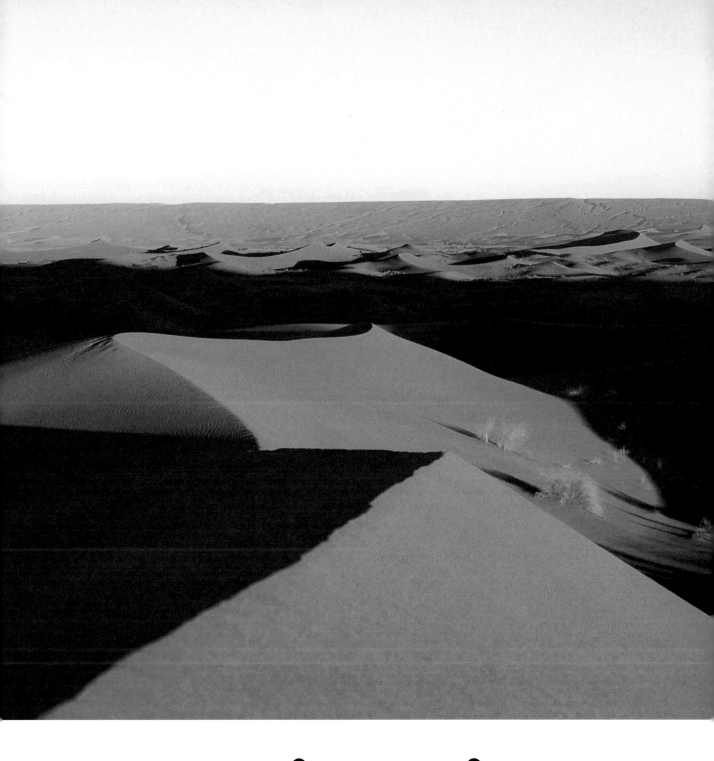

Fascinating

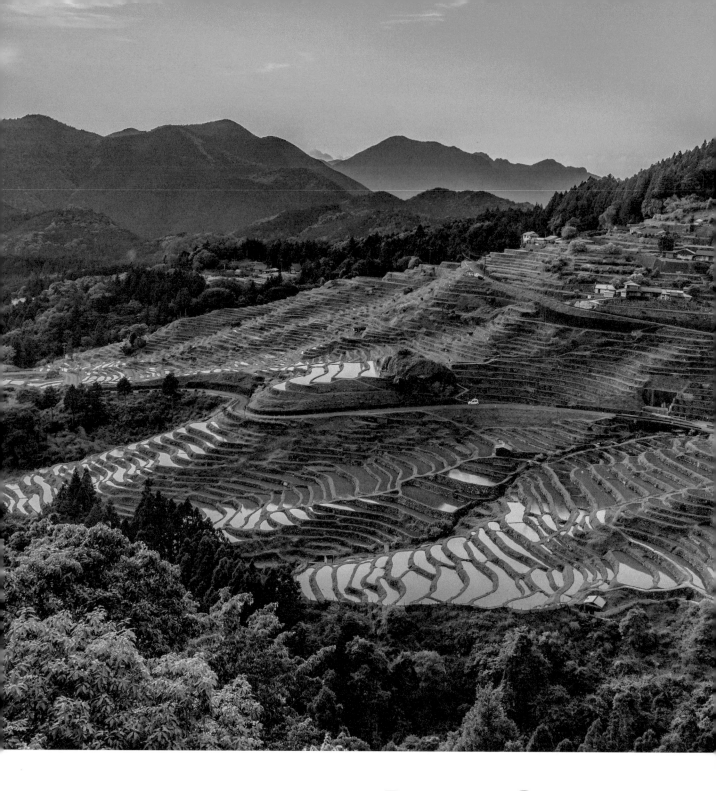

Wonderful

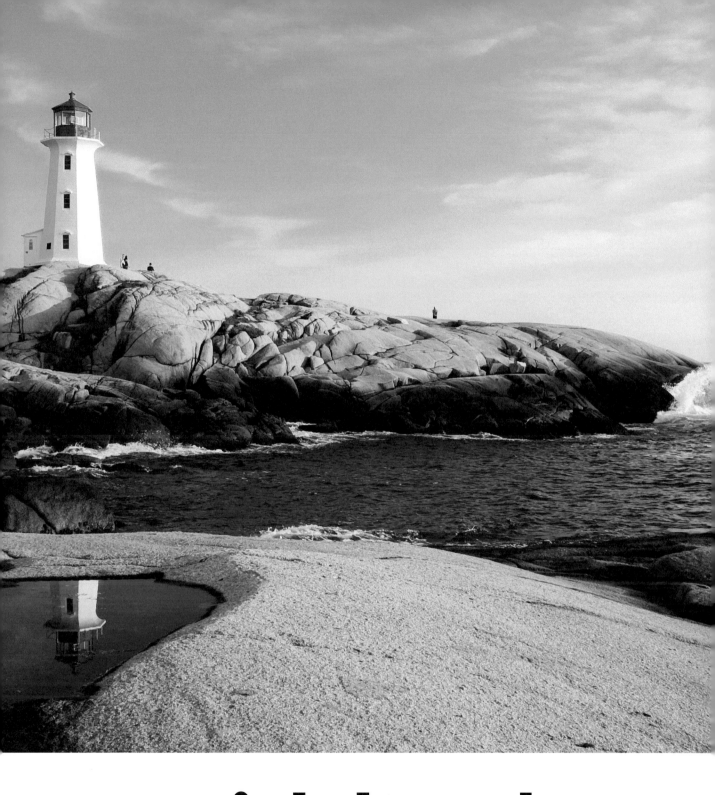

Laid-back

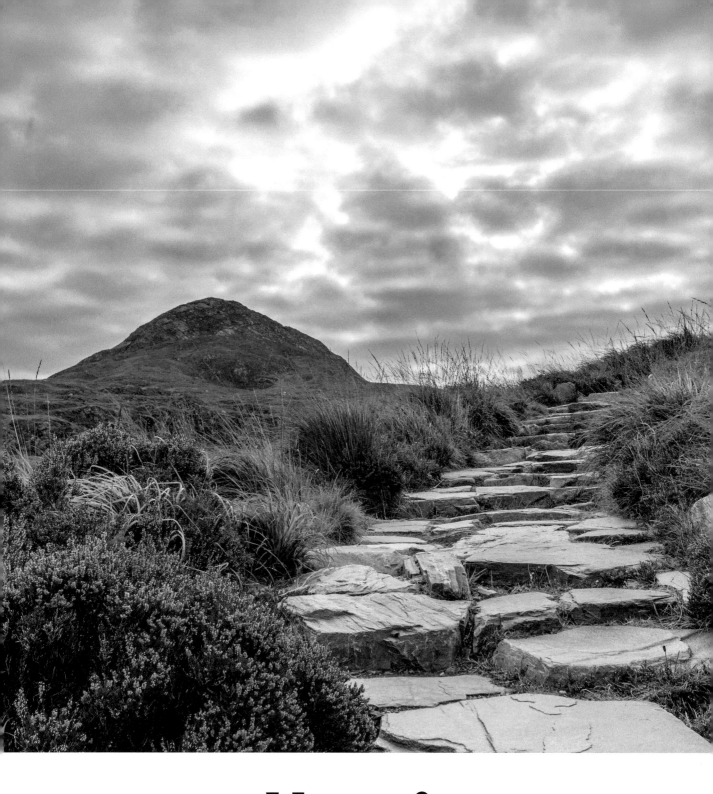

Alluring

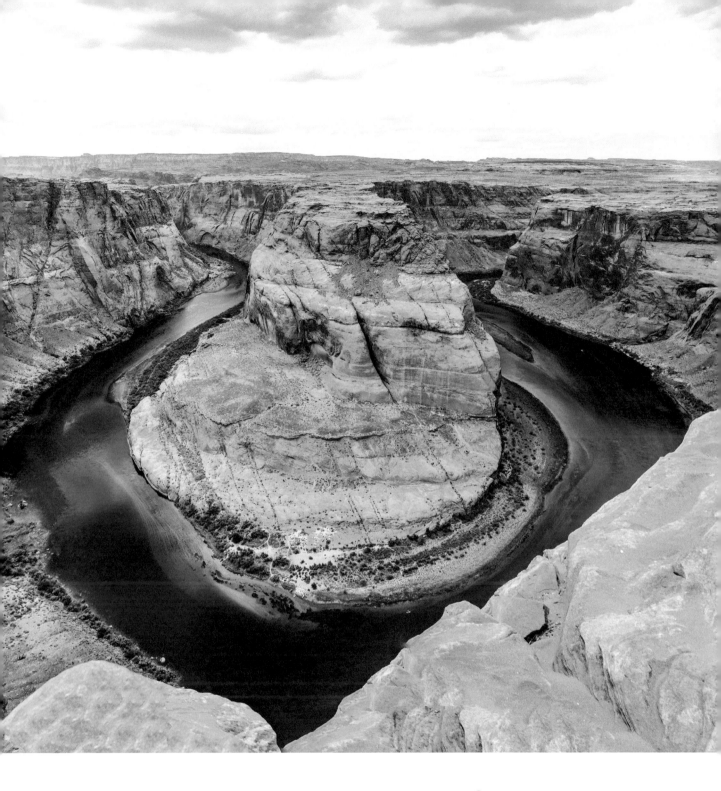

Splendid

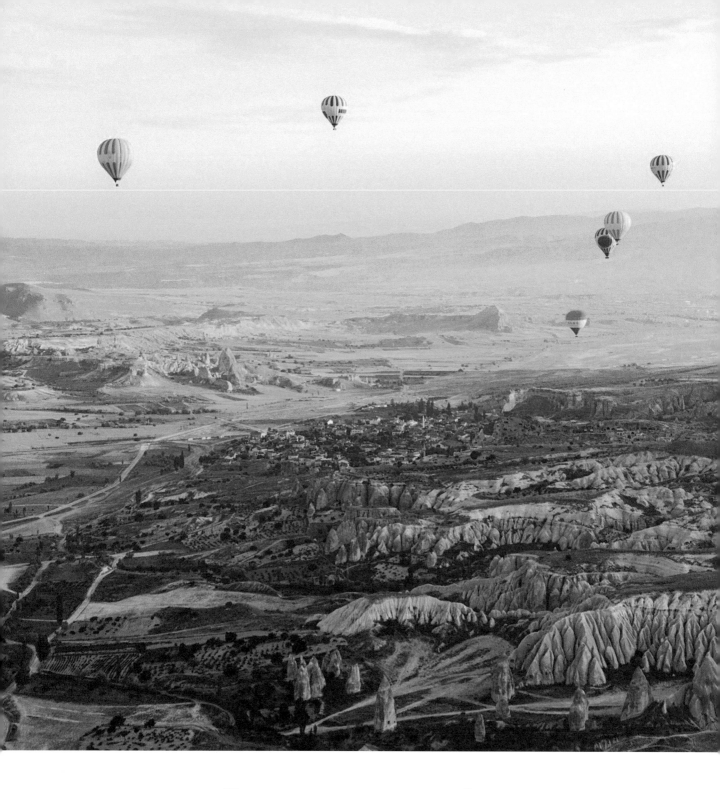

Charming

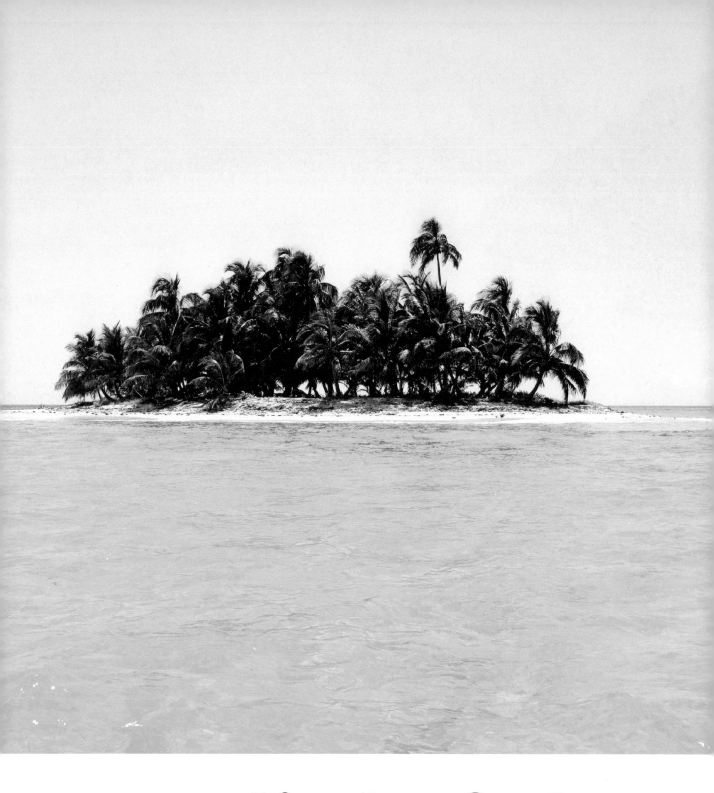

Delightful

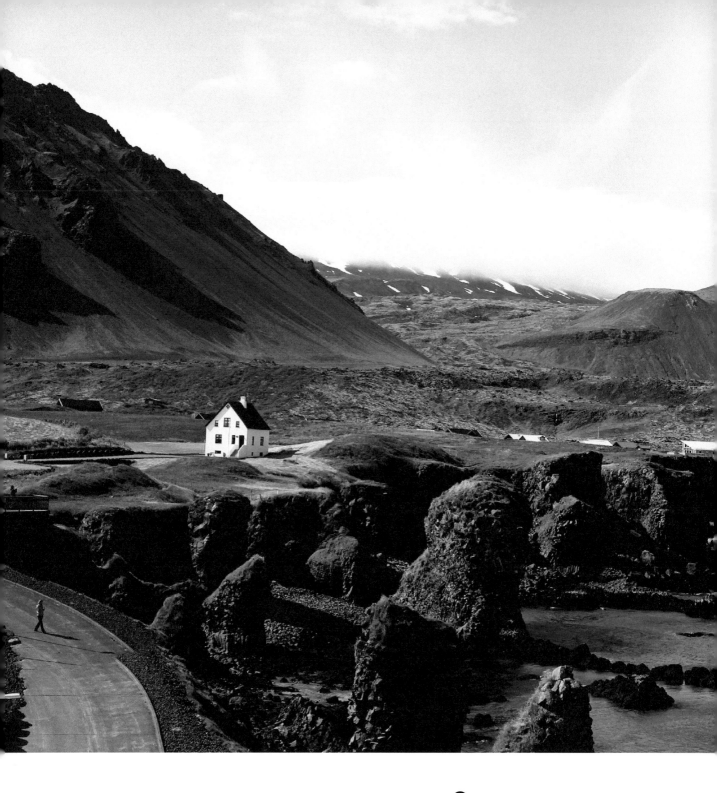

Sanguine

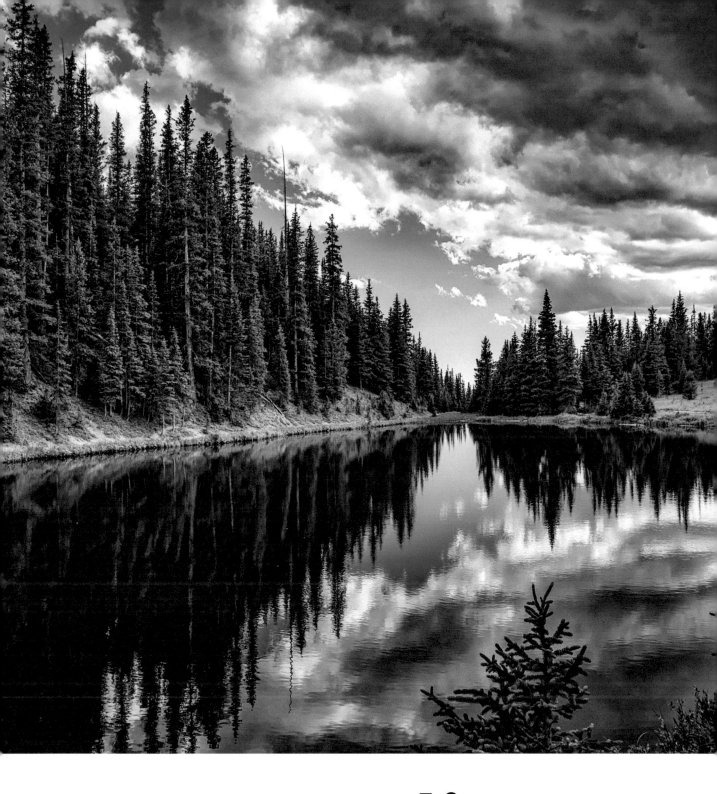

Appealing

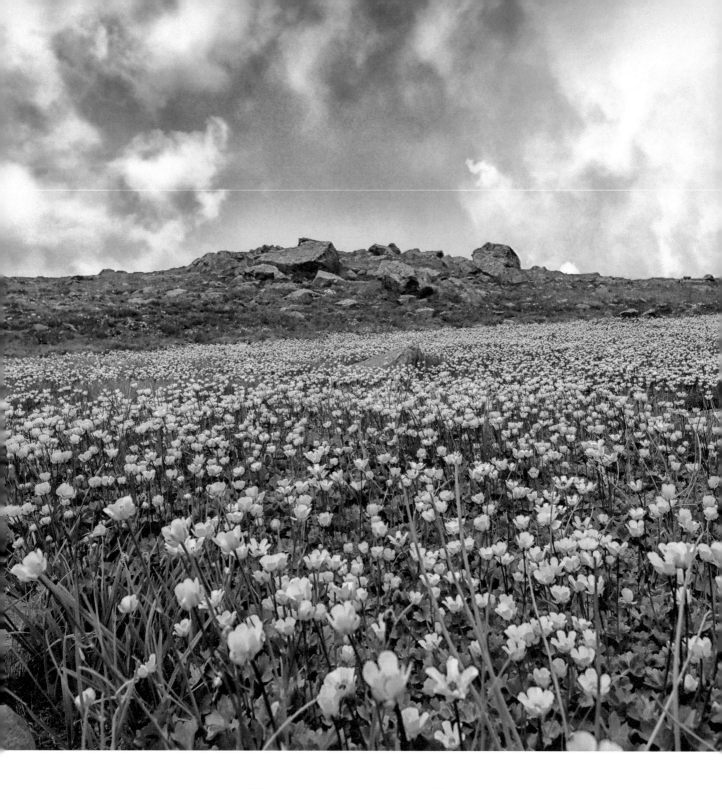

Pleasing

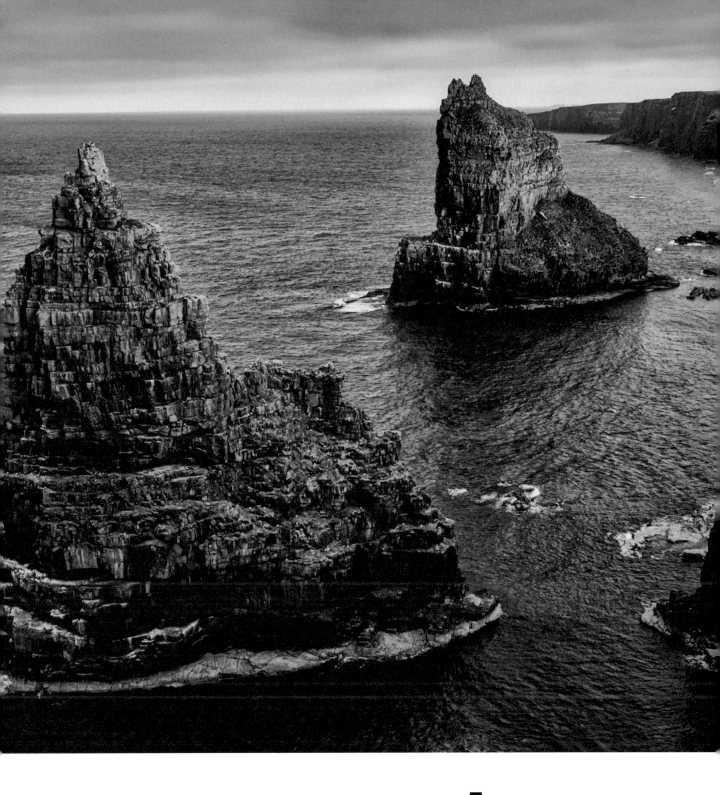

Grand

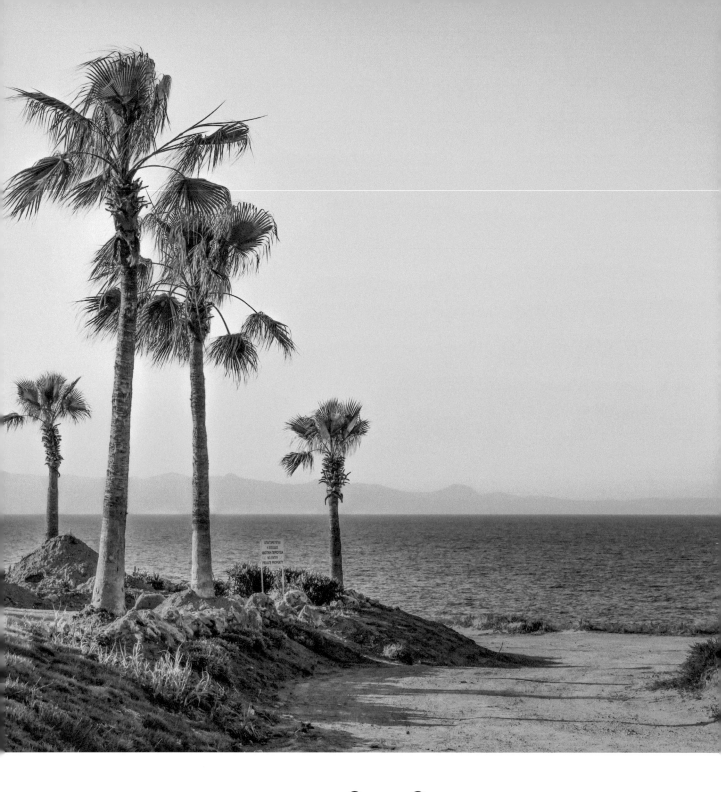

Inviting

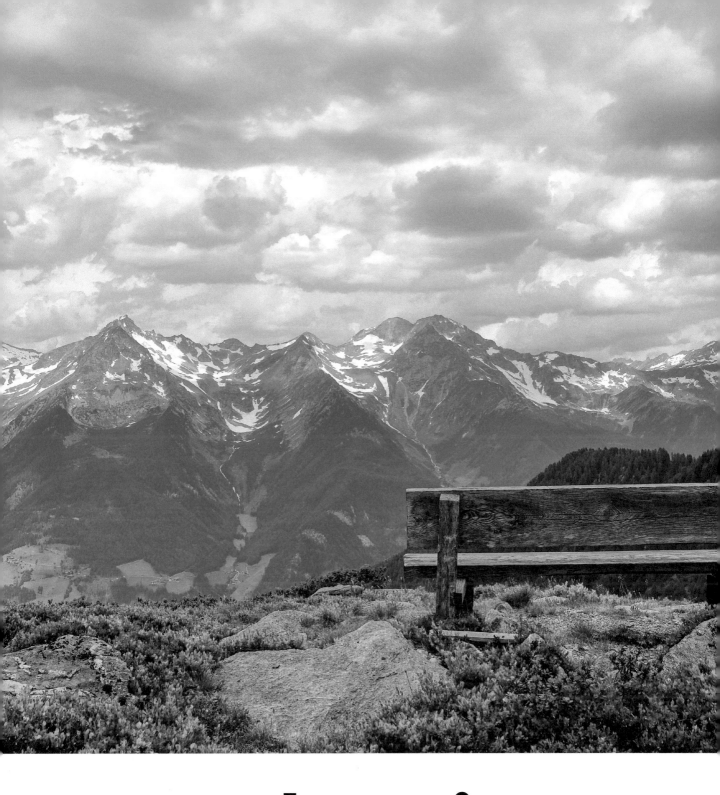

Beckoning

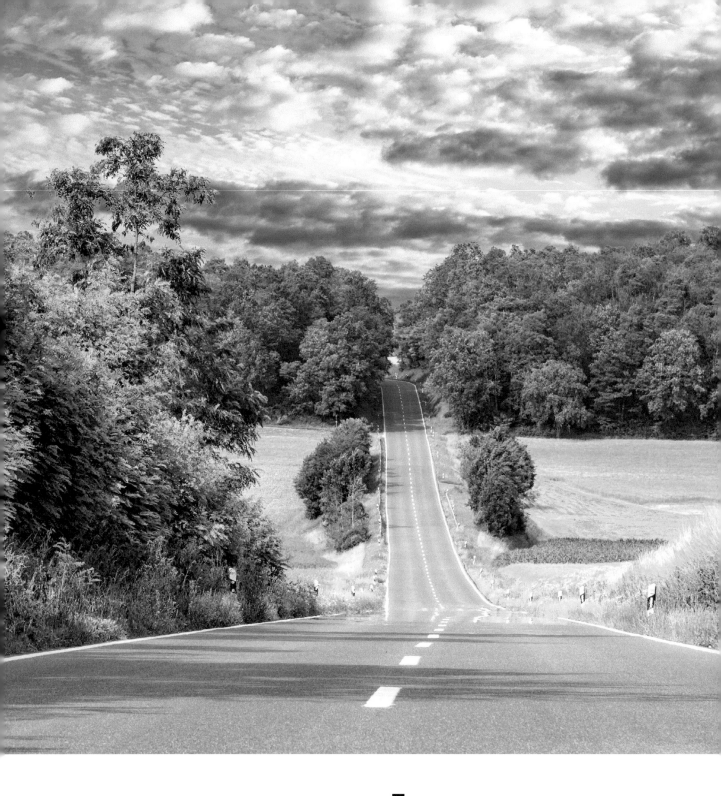

Wondrous

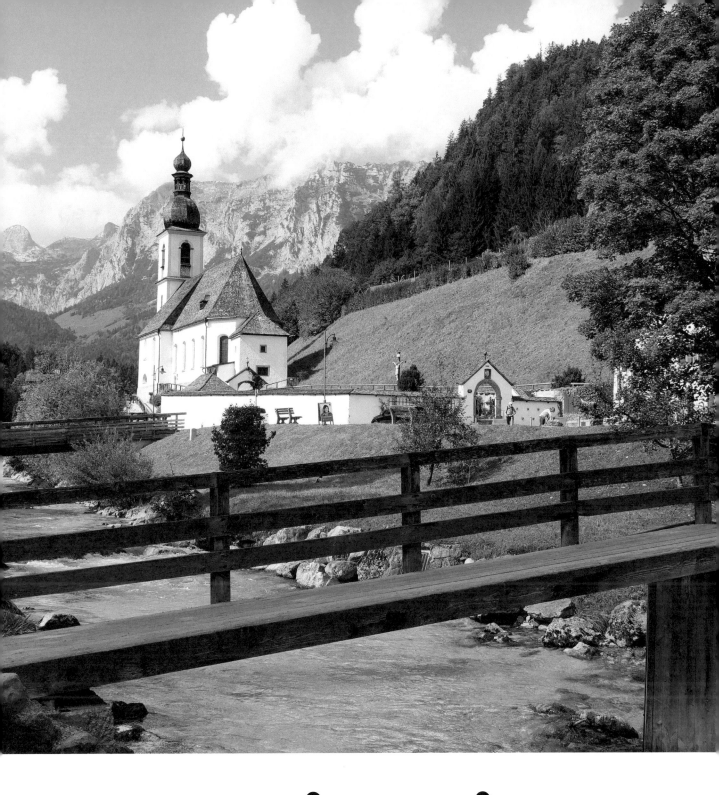

Captivating

Breathtaking

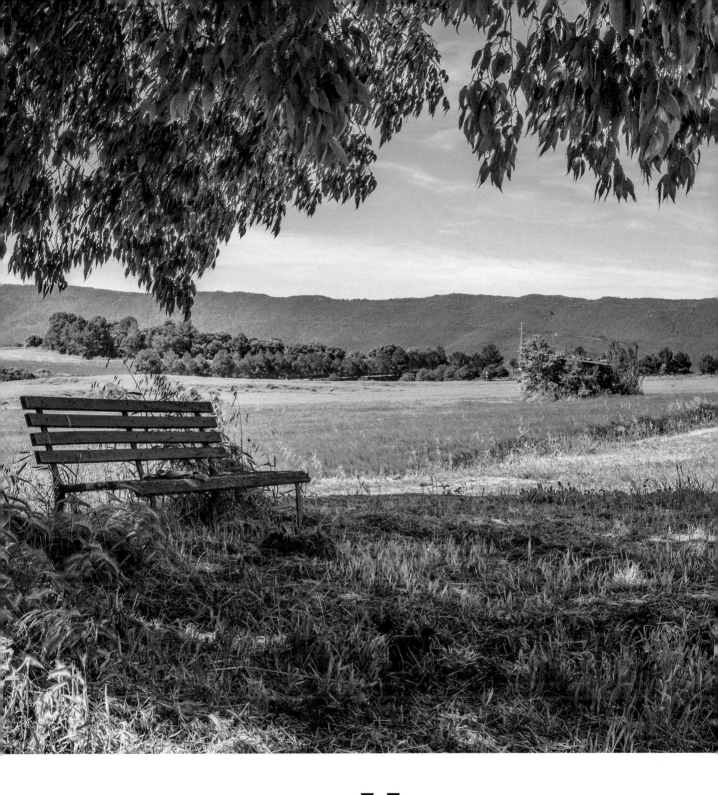

Excellent

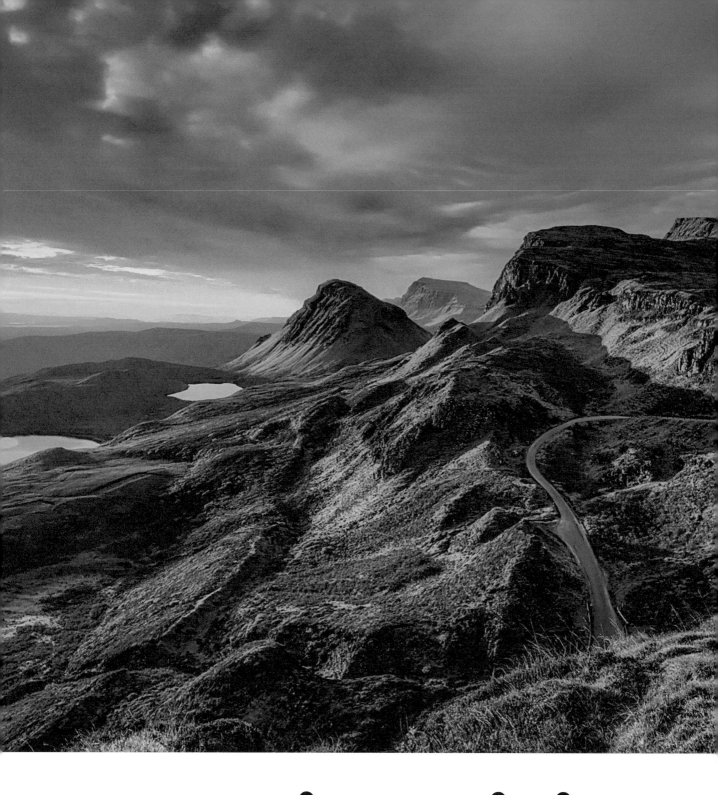

Awe-inspiring

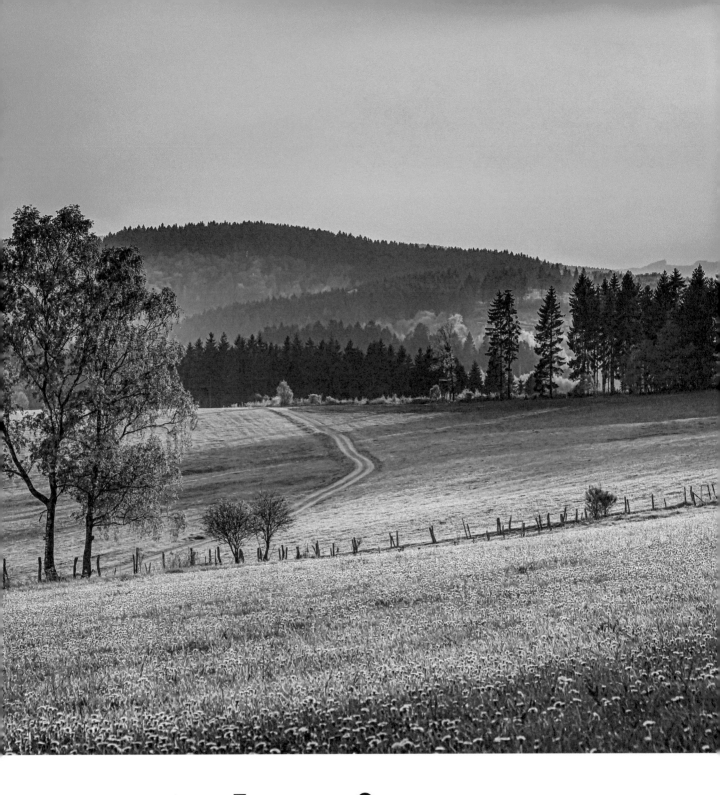

Glorious

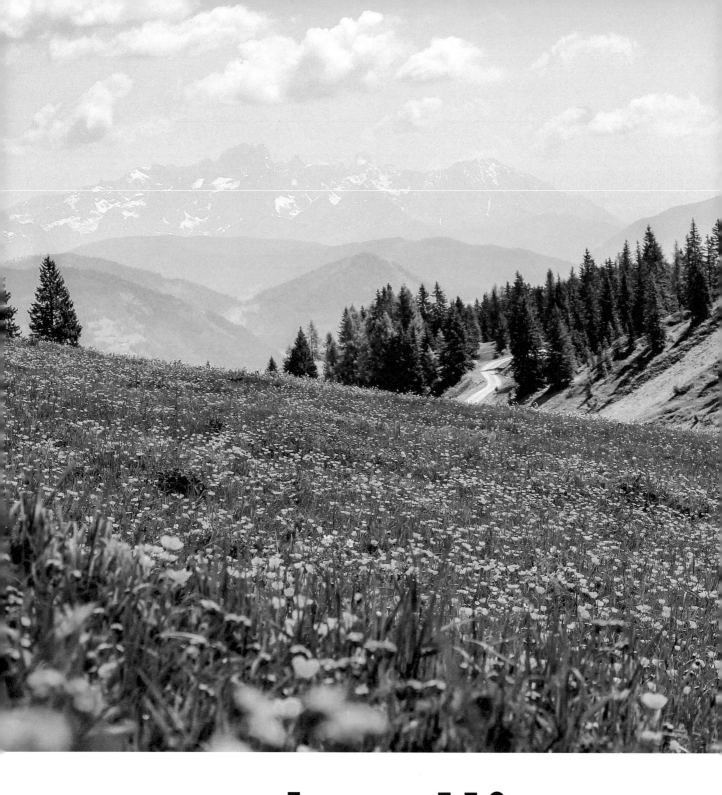

Enthralling

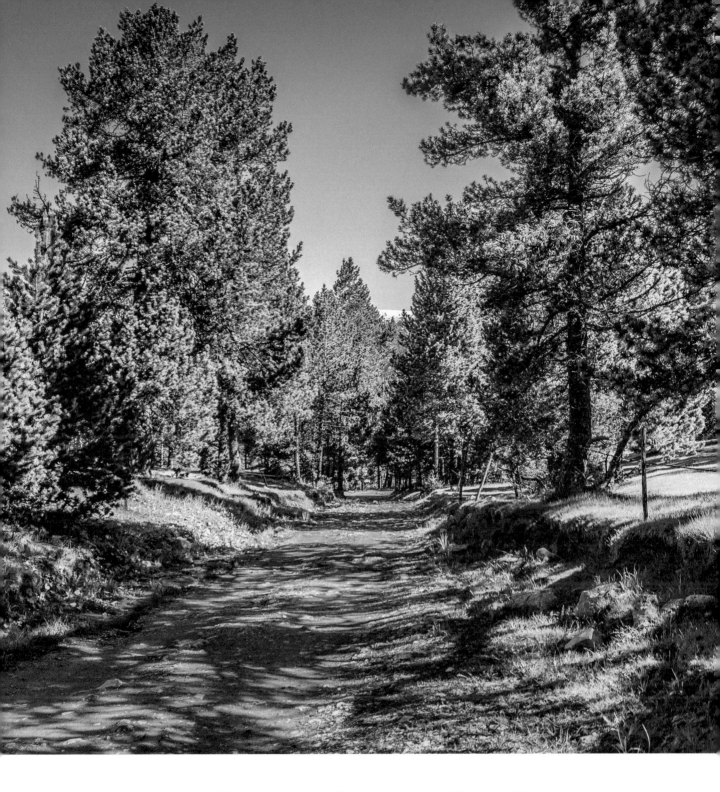

Admirable

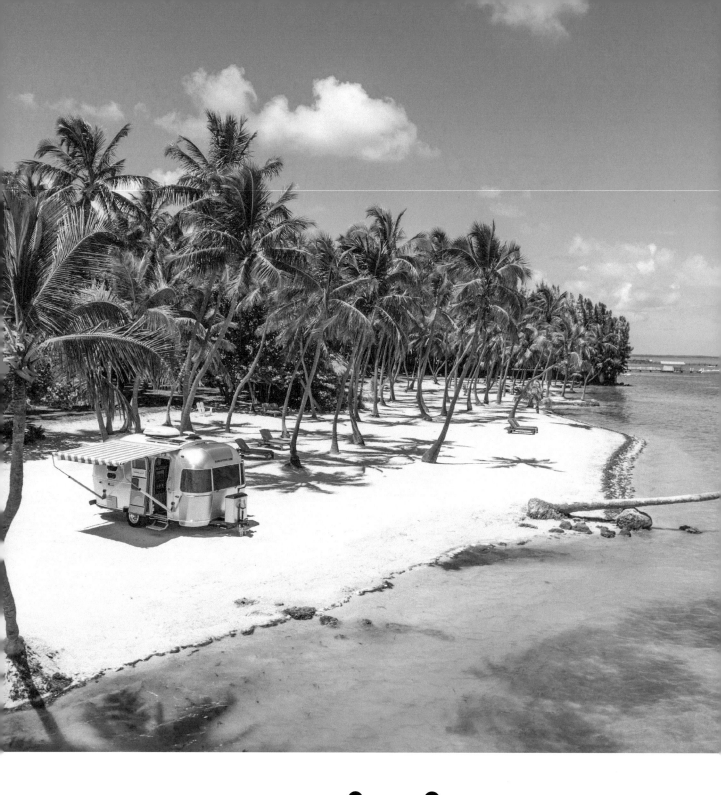

Enticing

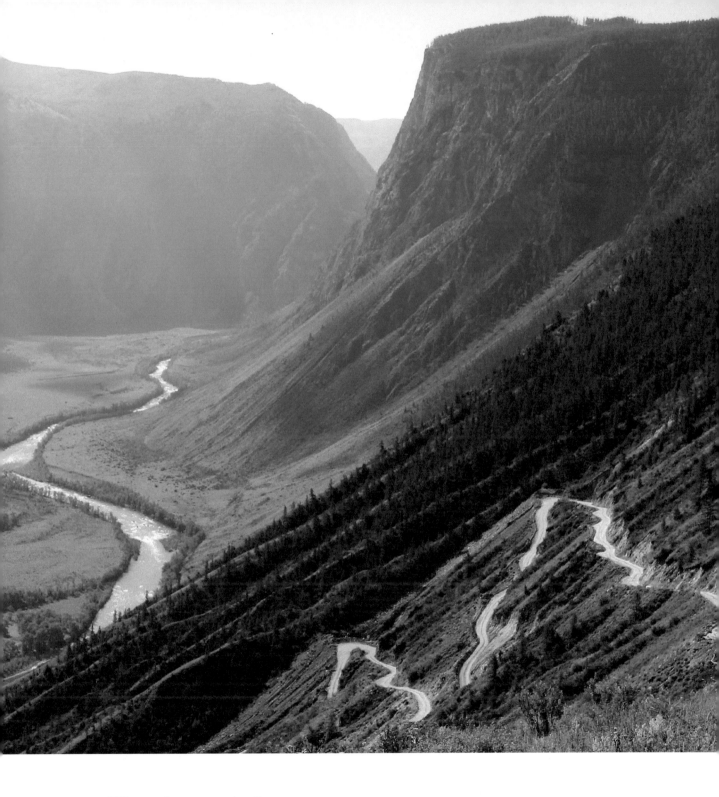

Statuesque

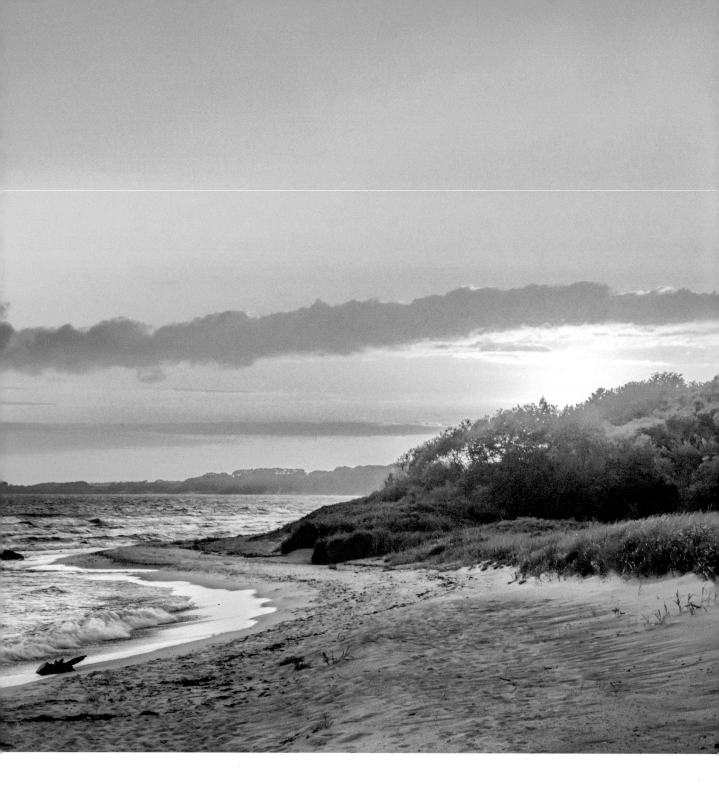

Pretty

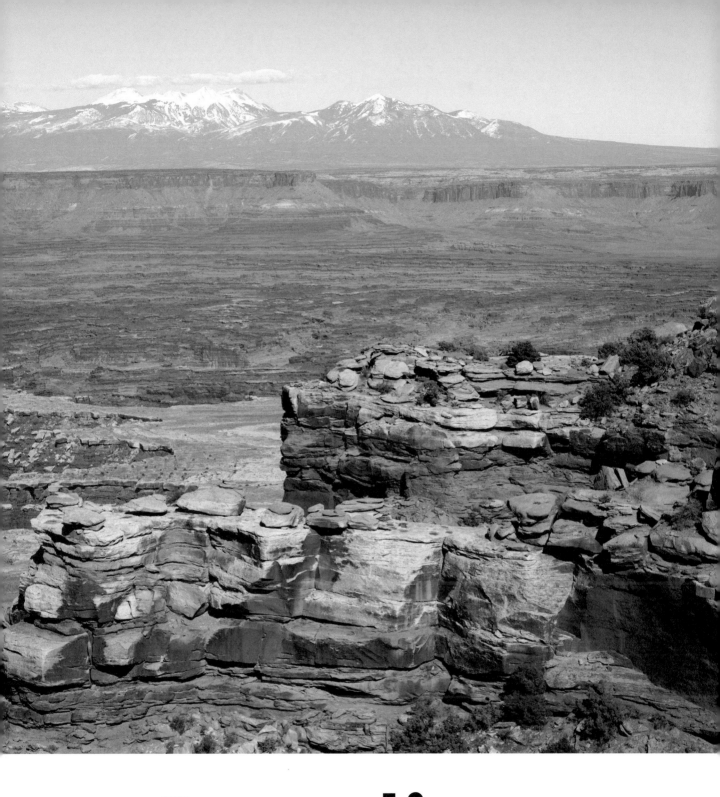

Dazzling

Sublime

Made in United States
Troutdale, OR
01/05/2024

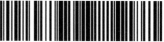

16715438R00026